My Prayers are with you. Please continue to pray for me. —Auburn W

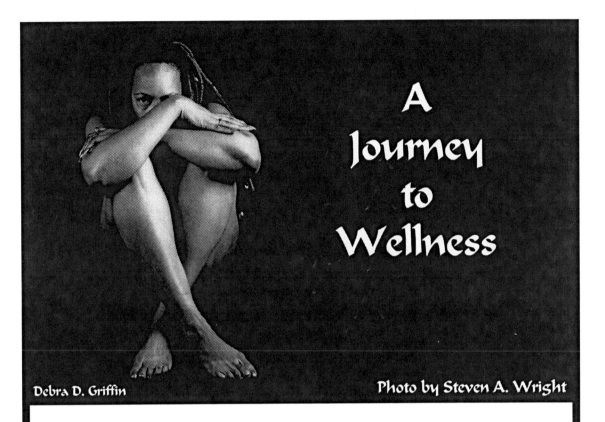

A Series of Collective Thoughts
by
Debra D. Griffin

© Copyright 2007 Debra D. Griffin

All rights reserved.
No republication of this material, in any form or medium,
is permitted
without express permission of the author.

ISBN# 978-0-9798217-2-1

First Edition First Printing
Printed in the United States of America
Candalyse Publishing Bethel, New York
www.CandalysePublishing.com

Cover Photo

Patti Dietrick

Book Cover Design

Donna Osborn Clark

Photography

Debra D. Griffin

Roy Gilliam

Steven A. Wright

Dr. Marcel Daniels

Nya Griffin-Ulibarri

Editor

R. M. Green

A Few Words From the Author

Born number nine of ten children to Reverend Jesse and Frances Mitchell, I was very shy and unable to speak my mind. It wasn't until I was forty-five years old and had taken a series of Photography classes that I found my voice. Having always wanting to write a book as I have a great love of poetry, it wasn't until the cancer that felt I had something important enough to write about.

To be able to have a window of opportunity and do what you love most is a blessing granted by God. Honest, it has been a pleasure to render this set of circumstances to render to you the words, which speak so vehemently in my heart.

I hope you enjoy my life's story. Please pray that the Lord continues to bless my family and me.

Debra

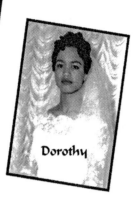
Dorothy

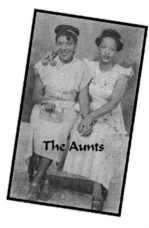
The Aunts

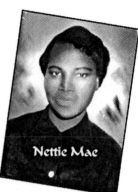
Nettie Mae

This collection of thoughts is dedicated to the memory of:
My sister-Dorothy L. Mitchell Bradley, my cousins-Chenetta Cage and Nettie Mae Mitchell, and to my Aunts-Maggie Mae Palmer and Nettie Mae Weatherspoon.

Your fight has not gone unnoticed. You are the driving force that moves me when the fight gets rough.

...And to Marva Mitchell who stood victoriously in her fight. Breast Cancer will be eradicated, one breast at a time.

Deb

Photos by Unknown Photographers

Although the idea of keeping a journal was Michele's at Breast Friends; I have taken both poetic and pictorial licenses hoping to make this project my own. Prior to her suggestion, the idea of writing down my thoughts each day throughout this tedious process did not occur to me. I had seen very few journals and the standard "Today I felt so bad that I kicked my dog" type of thing was a real turn off to me.

Also, I had never kept a journal and I did not know where to begin. Michele suggested going back to the last place I felt whole. So I did. Thank you, Michele.

Writing in this journal helped me, I hope reading it helps you.

"What you do after you are diagnosed with breast cancer will determine your outcome."

Revonia J. Truby

These are very powerful words that have a very sobering effect. Words, that if taken to heart can be used to fight by. Words, that if properly received can be used to live by. These words gave me a choice, and I chose to fight for life.

As I was trying to figure out my role in this screenplay that was literally becoming my life, I took these words into prayer. That evening I told God I didn't know what to do, but I would follow him wherever he led me. That night I only knew this: I could not do it alone. Not without my Lord and not without my friends and family.

Once armed with need to reflect and the need to document the fight, it was here I believe my journey began.

Reflections

The following journal entries are but a few of the thoughts which occurred to me, and were written just days after my diagnosis of breast cancer. At this point it became clear to me that I had something to say. That I was carrying around some real pain that needed to be exorcized and I started to write with a vengeance.

The death of my childhood sweetheart and the divorce from spouse were two issues that I thought I had dealt with. Life goes on but pain if not eradicated is ravenous.

BEFORE KHAFID

Debra D. Griffin

Photo by Roy Gilliam

My life before Khafid was simple and honest. I spent most of my days working and the evenings I spent at home with the girls.

On the weekends we would most often be found walking the boardwalk at Venice Beach or visiting one of the local amusement parks.

We were a close lot of a strange sort sharing everything but our pain. We never spoke about our loss. We never cried aloud.

Daughters

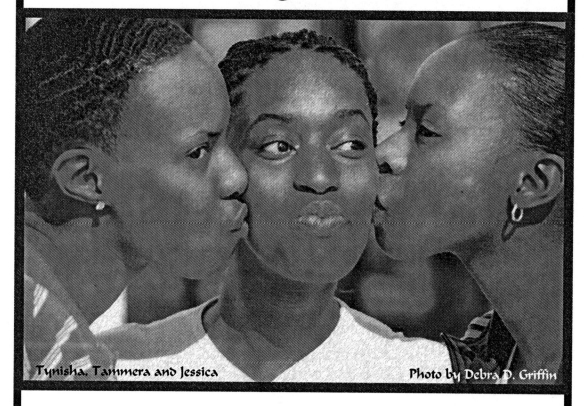

Tynisha, Tammera and Jessica
Photo by Debra D. Griffin

All that I am,
All that I will ever be,
Is because,
You are.

It is only now that I am able to measure the contrast between living healthy and merely existing. When one lives she or he celebrates the simple milestones which life has to offer. The birth of a child or even the day to day care of that child becomes the grand focus and you are able not only to see, but to revel in its payoffs.

Retrospectively, I can also see that even after losing my spouse I had a multitude of reasons to be thankful for - Tammera, Tynisha and Jessica, my daughters.

"loneliness"

Debra D. Griffin

Photo by Roy Gilliam

There were many things that I discovered while I was trying to learn to do for myself and the girls.

Many things, but if asked I would have to say it was the way I dealt with loneliness which surprised me the most.

I was bad at it and it haunted me. At that time there wasn't anything or anyone that could make it palatable to me. Yet, I dined at its table and consumed it's misery.

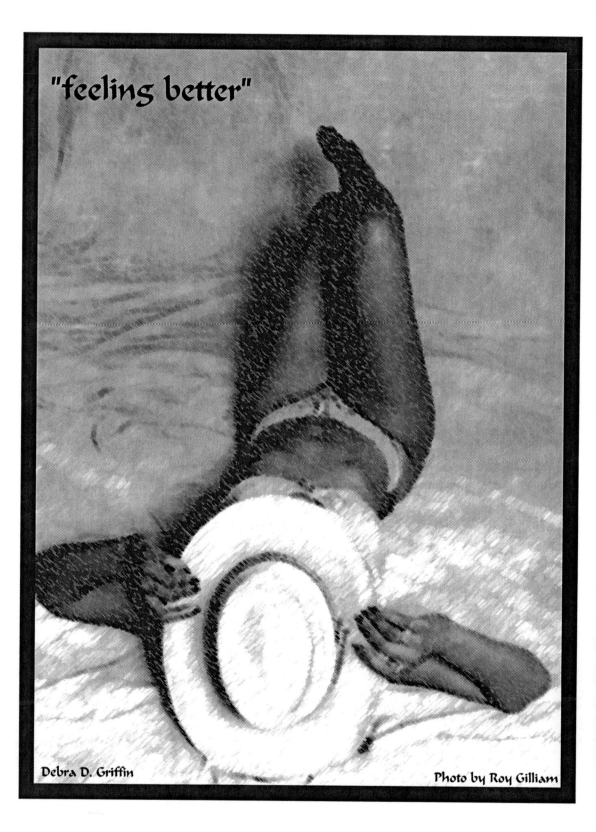
"feeling better"

Debra D. Griffin

Photo by Roy Gilliam

It is said that time heals all wounds. Yet, Mother Time wasn't as gracious where I was concerned, for she only saw fit to mask my woes.

Feeling better I stepped out into the world and found companionship or now I'm left to wonder if it wasn't companionship who found me.

At any rate, the fact is that I did meet (and for whatever reason or how clouded my judgement was) I did marry Mr. Khafid A. Ibrahim.

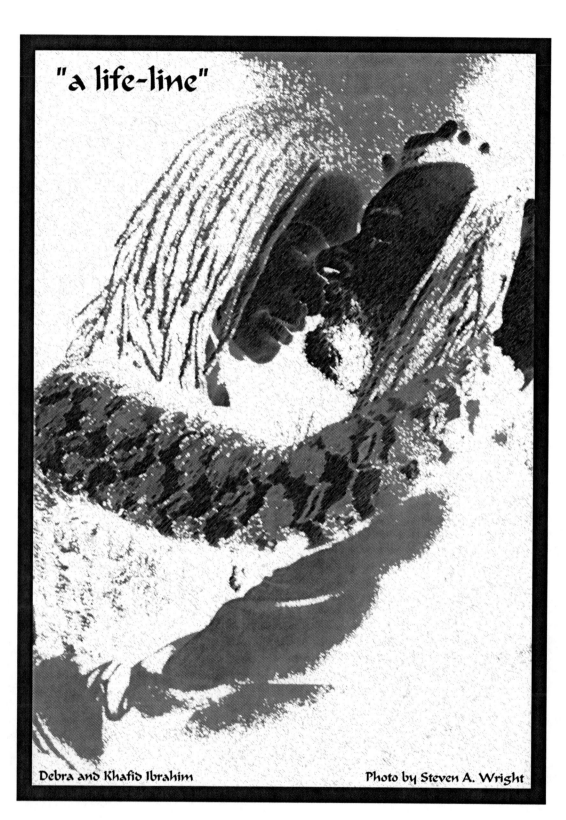

"a life-line"

Debra and Khafid Ibrahim

Photo by Steven A. Wright

In all honesty I have to admit that when I found Khafid I was both broken and torn. The day he came walking into my life it wasn't quite two years after my husband's death.

Khafid offered me a life-line and being the drowning soul that I was I took it. Hook, line and sinker, I took it.

Now with that being said let me also say that nothing I had experienced prior to our meeting prepared me for what lay in wait for me.

No one I had ever known or met had ever been so cruel or mean to me. Until then I had been the cherished child of Reverend Jesse E. Mitchell and Beloved wife of Marvin Griffin.

Please understand that I don't fault Khafid for my illness, I merely note his arrival as the last memory I have of my own personal sense of being whole.

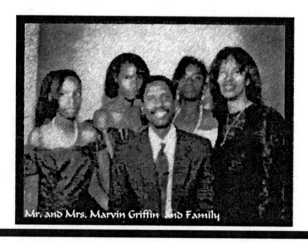

Mr. and Mrs. Marvin Griffin and Family

Photographer Unknown

Khafid brought with him few gifts - his four children that he fathered with two other women were the most valued presents I received.

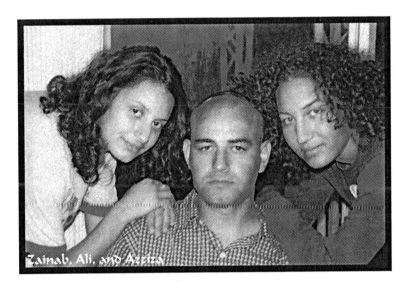

There will always be a joy in my heart, merely mention the names, Azziza, Ali, Zainab and Stewart.

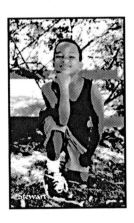

Photos by Debra D. Griffin

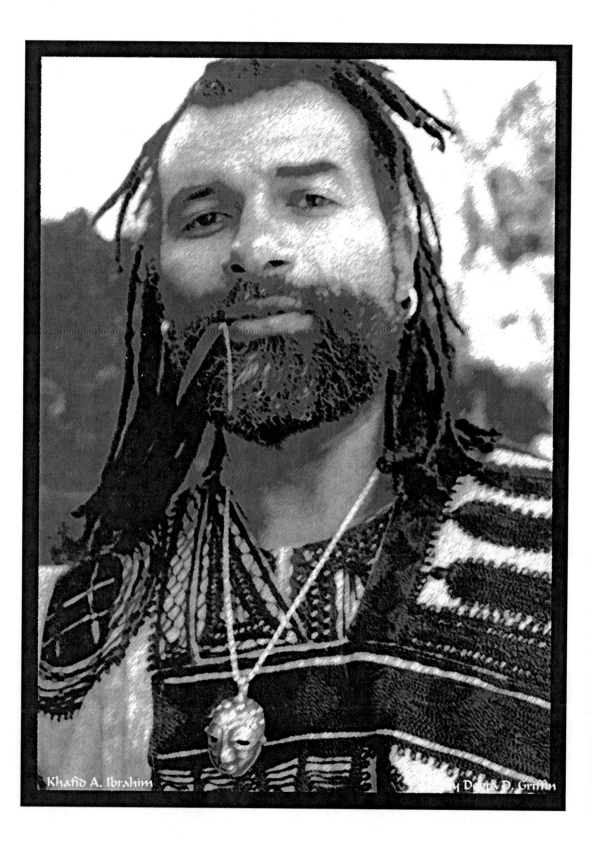

I believe Mr. Ibrahim to be a sociopath and I was just one of his many would-be victims. I also believe that if not for my great sense of God and self I would not have been able to make it in his world of lies, deceit and dishonor.

Believe me I do not have the need to punish Khafid for his behavior which lead to the erosion of our marriage. Nor do I have the need to hide those facts from the historical pages of my life. We live in a country where 50% of our marriages fail. A great number of them fail due to adultery. The facts are simple. I went to bed one night in the loving arms of my husband and I woke the next morning to learn that I had been sleeping with the community penis.

Now I don't understand many things so it shouldn't come to a big surprise that I don't understand, why a man with so much to lose would gamble on his marriage only to gain what he can balance on the tip of his phallus. Nothing!

Sometimes life is hard at best. Even today I am surprised by the many accomplishments that God blessed and bestowed on me during that time. As I was able to graduate with a credential in Photography, find my niece Linda who had been relinquished to adoption, and travel both Europe and Africa. Now you go figure.

It wasn't until I had nowhere to call home that I started entertaining the idea of divorce. Khafid got into an argument with the landlord and we were evicted.

The toll that heart break and stress plays on the body can sometimes be too much. So looking for relief I sought the comfort of a good friend. Food.

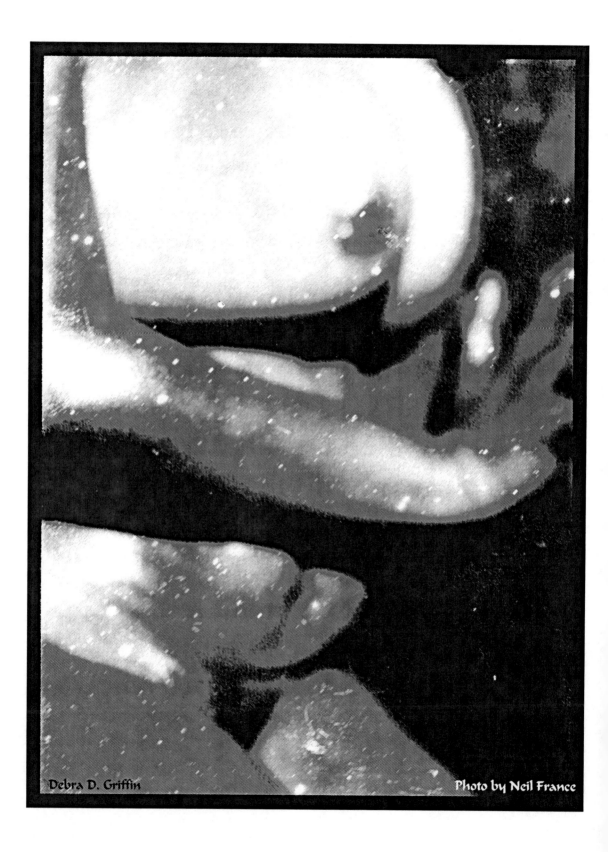

To hear the phrase, "He drank me and I ate him" roll off the tip of my tongue floored me. Yet it had to be said as this phrase, for me, marked the day I knew I was fragmented and needed to be whole.

It was on this day I left Khafid and on this day I could see peace of mind in view. Yes I weighted in at a whopping 219 pounds. Yes, and shortly afterwards my list of medical problems started to accumulate. High cholesterol, high blood pressure and poor circulation plagued me. Yes, I was ill, yet there was a joy on the horizon for me.

The Journey

"at Life's Shores"

Nya at Catalina Island Shore

Photo by Debra D. Griffin

A Journey to Wellness

To be well. To be free from illness. Now this may be an elusive dream, however, I find myself swimming through a vast sea of illness trying to emerge unscathed at life's shores.

Just to be, to be whole again is my current struggle in this watery depth.

Lord please keep me afloat long enough to plant my feet on solid ground.

A FIGHT FOR WELLNESS

Global Cardio Care Staff Member

Photo by Debra D. Griffin

After loosing about 50 pounds on the Atkins Diet (which also exacerbated my chief medical complaints) I noticed that my level of fatigue went unchanged. I could only walk a matter of a few yards before my legs would burn like I ran a mile. It was then that I sought help and was referred to Global Cardio Care.

Once at Global I was diagnosed with Arteriosclerosis and I began my EECP Therapy. I saw a notable improvement right away and was able to take ownership in my progress.

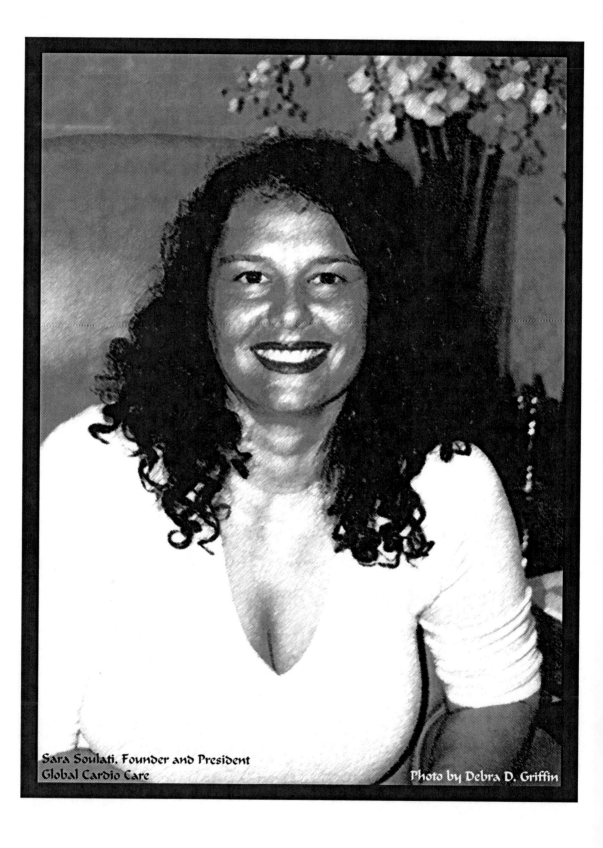

Global made this easy as I was taught and exposed to a great number of things there. Lets see, nutrition, balancing rest and exercise, the importance of drinking the proper amounts of water. I learned about herbs and colon cleansing, what role fibre plays on the body. I looked forward to my handouts.

Sara says....

I was encouraged to continue my journey to wellness and I knew that under their tutelage and guidance I could do it, I felt good, strong and both physically and mentally prepared.

Global's Staff Monitoring The Patient's Vitals

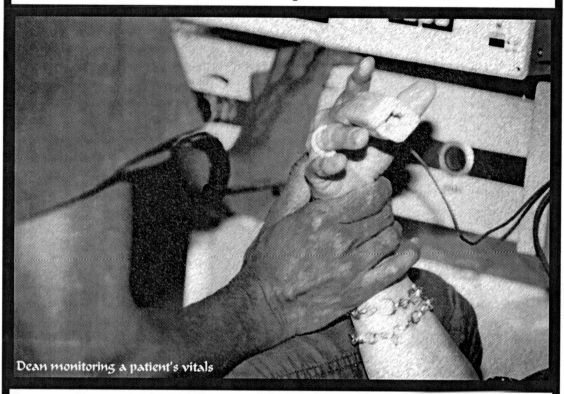

Dean monitoring a patient's vitals

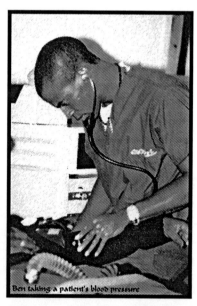

Ben taking a patient's blood pressure

Never will I forget the kindness I received from the staff at Global, they felt like home. The friendships made there I trust will be lasting. What a blessing to receive just what you need when times get hard. Healing hands and smiling faces!

Photos by Debra D. Griffin

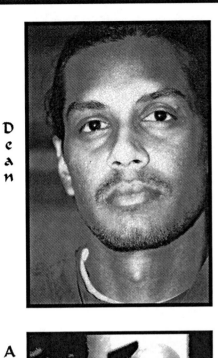
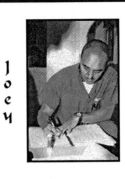
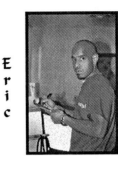
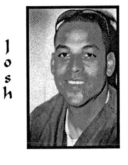
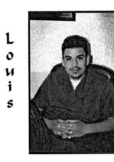

Global Cardio Care's Staff

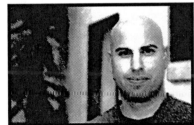
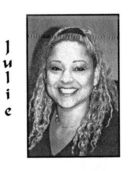
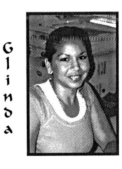
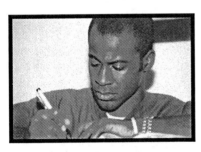
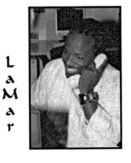
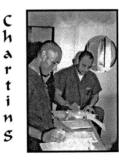
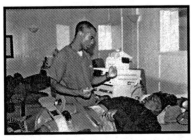

Photos by Debra D. Griffin

A Cancer Diagnosis

Tynisha R. Griffin

Photo by Debra D. Griffin

The first diagnosis to come along was not my own. My Tynisha was diagnosed with a brain tumor. Cancer. The phrase brain cancer will torment my soul throughout eternity. In fact I hear it's monstrous melodies resounding through my being as I recant it's utterance.

I can only imagine that my first conversation with God just moments after my arrival to heaven will be about cancer of the brain.

Lord help me as I am your child.

There is no greater fear that a woman can experience. Nothing, Not A Thing will ever compare to the pure unadulterated hell that is felt when a mother is confronted with the possibility of losing a child. No matter how old or what the reason, the threat of losing her baby is just totally unbearable.

I want to tell you that God will make a way for you, he will keep his devine promise. The thing that would have been too much for me to bear he has bound and taken from me.

My sweet young woman lives.

Tye's Tumor

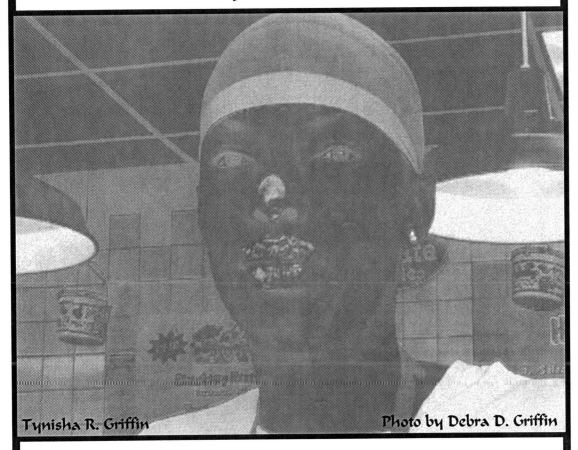

Tynisha R. Griffin

Photo by Debra D. Griffin

They performed a biopsy on Tye's tumor the day before Thanksgiving. She was also given a round of Chemo and Radiation. To date her tumor is unchanged and is not growing.

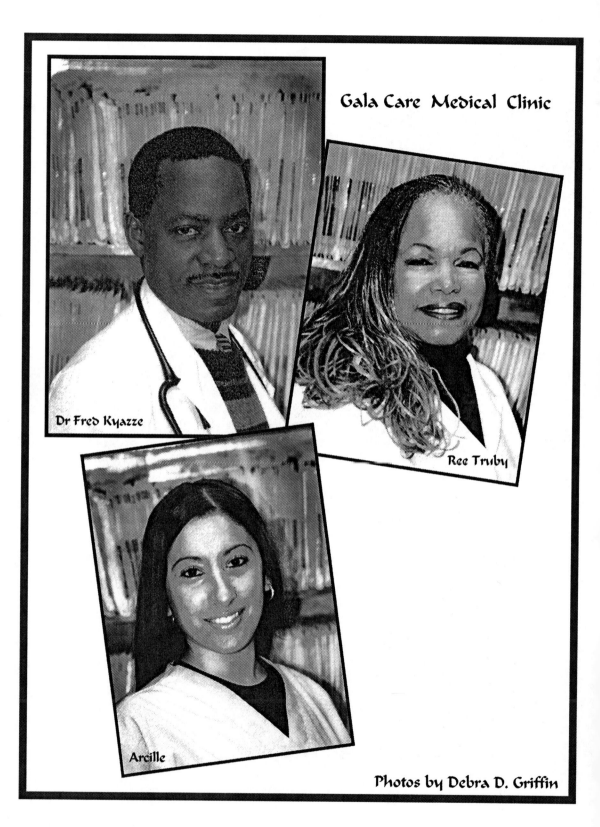

Now you know, Cancer should have been my biggest fear. I have Fibroid Cystic Breast, but the thing that led me to my primary care physician at Gala Care Medical Clinic was vanity. I was seeking a breast reduction. The weight loss left me too small to carry the large breast that yet remained. My posture had changed and the back aches were killing me.

I was seen by Ree Truby the Nurse Practitioner (Ree is also my big sister) who noticed the changes in my breast and asked Dr. Kyazze to have a look at them. I was referred to Long Beach MemorialCare Breast Center.

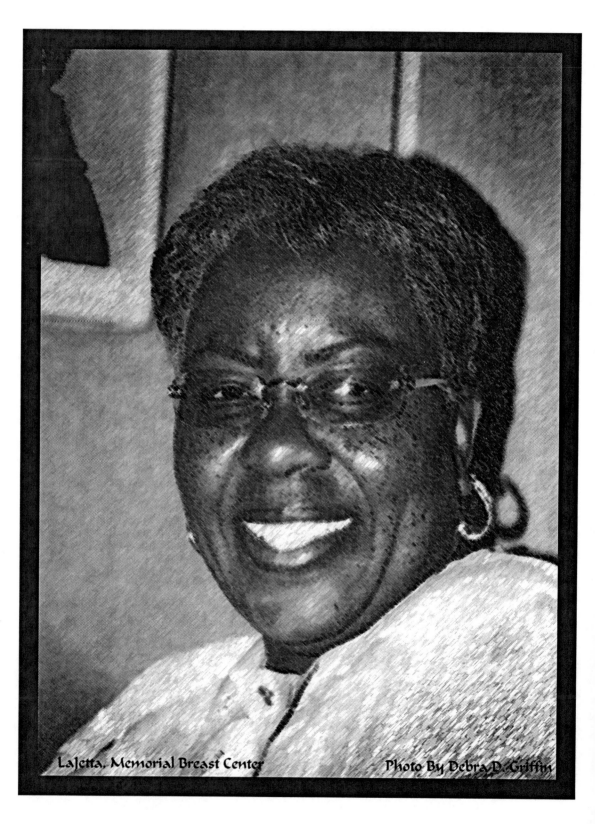

LaJetta, Memorial Breast Center   Photo By Debra D. Griffin

My visit to the Breast Center began like all the others. The clerk, LaJetta, checked me in and went over all of my insurance documentation. You know the drill.

I was called to the back and given a gown to change into. Shortly afterwards the Tech escorted me back into one of the mammogram stations and the testing began.

The next room I was invited to was for the ultrasound with the Radiologist. She also aspirated a few cysts.

Fear, Dr. Gretchen Stipec and I

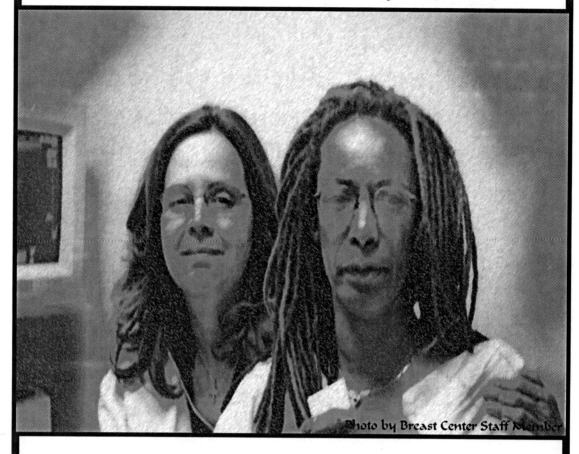

Photo by Breast Center Staff Member

It is impossible to express just how I was feeling on this day as words can only relay a certain portion of what the human brain can compose. But, if a picture paints a thousand words, then it is safe to say that fear was written all over my face.

The mammogram and ultrasound showed a rather large mass approximately four cm in diameter in the lower left quadrant of my left breast. The Radiologist performed a core biopsy and I was given a book on cancer. "THE CANCER BOOK."

I somehow managed to maintain composure until I got to my car, but as soon as I closed the door the tears began to flow and I cried and cried. I did wail like the chief mourner at a Baptist Funeral.

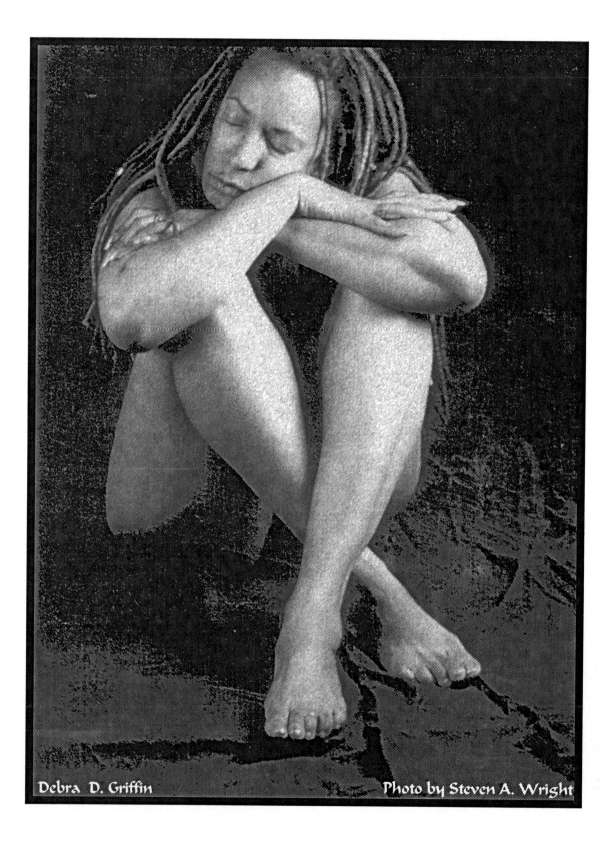

When I finally pulled myself together, I called a friend, Dean Dass, and told him about the test. He was working and could not get to me, but what he said to me was quite remarkable.

Dean told me that someone who loved me was already with me. I thought he was talking about God until he told me to put my arms around myself and hold on. He also said that no one could love me like I could.

So I held myself and when I felt better I started my car, said good-bye to my friend, and drove home.

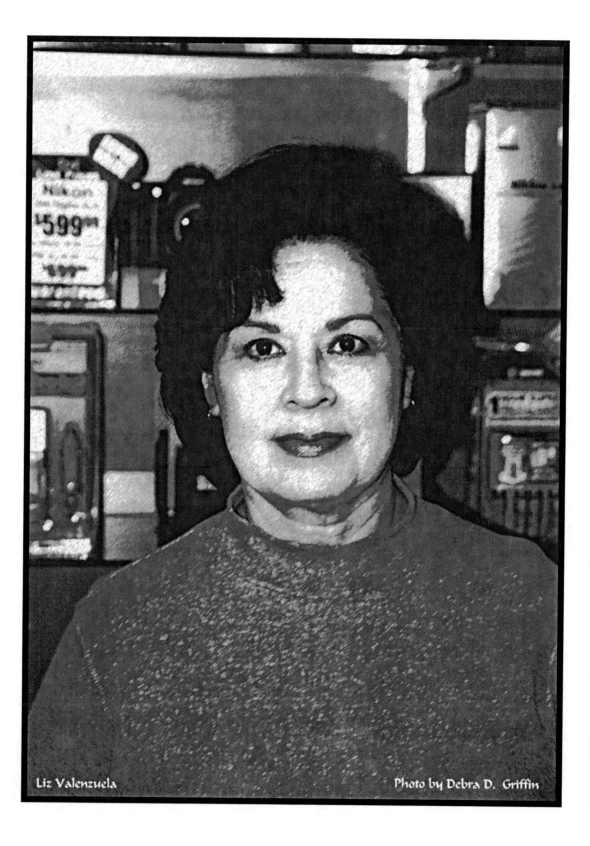

Liz Valenzuela Photo by Debra D. Griffin

I will never forget the day Dr. Stipec called to discuss the results of my core biopsy. I was at work alone. Funny thing is that Liz, my friend and boss, just announced she was going on a break. She never takes a standard away break (a quick trip to the backroom for personal reflection is more her style).

At any rate, I received the call and listened as closely as possible while Dr. Stipec gently filled my ears with medical terminology. But this is what I heard her to say, "Girl you are going to die!!! And the thing that is going to kill you has a name."
Invasive Ductal Carcinoma

Just the word cancer is a very frightening thing and God knows that I've had more than my fair share of loss due to this vicious monster who attacks from within. Who's victims are left mere shells of themselves awaiting death to bring relief from it's mighty grip. I thought of Dorothy.

And as tears of self pity and my new reason to re-mourn my losses strolled down my face a customer walked into the store and my attention shifted to her needs.

I waited on her and when she walked out the door I never felt more alone.

Once Liz returned from her brake I dialed one of the numbers the doctor had given me. A woman named Michele answered. She introduced me to her organization, Breast Friends, and gave me what seemed like mountains of information. She knew I needed to be pointed in the right direction and was eager to help.

There are two pieces of info I came away with from that conversation with Michele that would be life saving. The Idea of keeping a journal and the telephone number to Breastlink. I did not know it then, but God was paving a path for me and all I needed to do was follow it. Thank-you Michele.

I don't know how but I finished my shift. Sometimes you just do what you have to do without thought. This is a good thing, at least it was on that day. Once I got home I called Ree and I told her.

She knew when she sent me to the the breast clinic what I was up against and was ready to guide me through this maze of decisions. I told her that Michele had given me a referral to see Dr. John Link at Breastlink. Turns out my sister worked with John years ago. She actually helped him setup the Oncology Department over at Long Beach Memorial Hospital.

Ree made an appointment for me.

Then we talked until she was sure we had covered everything I needed to know about breast cancer and its treatment. The old, the new and the experimental.

While we waited for the appointment with Link she took me to see a surgeon, Dr. Tomi Evans. There we planned what we were going to do after Chemo and/or radiation.

Ree promised she would never leave me. I asked her to tell me about the day I was born. Turns out my sweet sister baked a cake to welcome me home. I felt her love as her memories flooded my heart. It was then I took a cleansing breath and fell in love with her all over again.

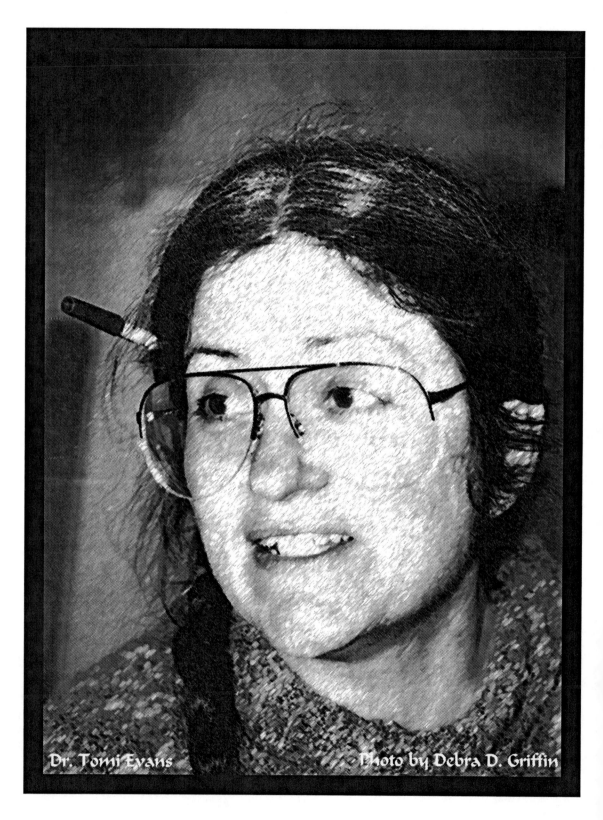

I found Dr. Evans to be a very delightful woman. She had a certain something that I was instantly drawn to, that thing which allows you to feel at home under the worst times. As she spoke to Ree and I, I could not help but to think, how very proud I was to be her patient. As she proved to be very strong and intelligent.

We three women sat and decided what would be our course of action. At this meeting we collectively determined that a bi-lateral mastectomy was necessary. We also talked about reconstruction and other choices. I was then referred to Dr. Marcel Daniels.

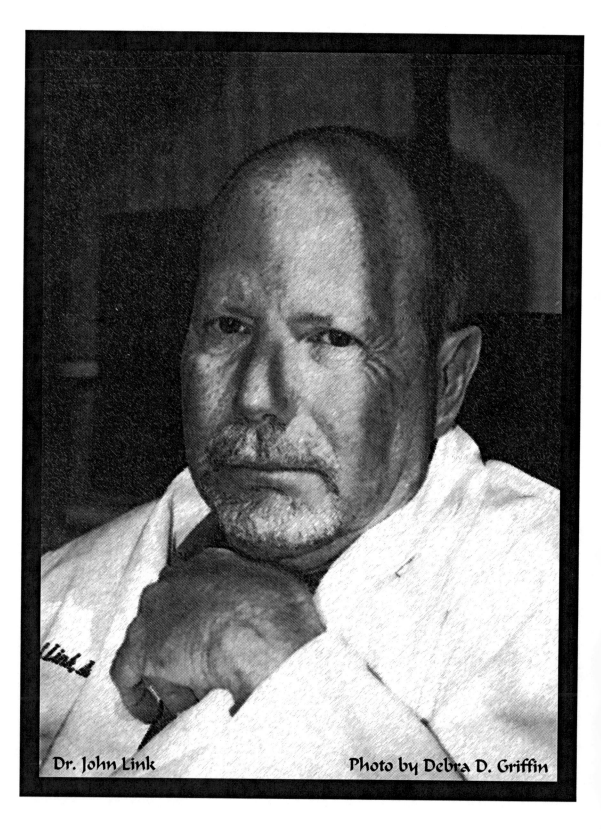

The Bible says, "Thou shalt not have any Gods before me." So just let me take this time to give praises to my heavenly father who has brought me along way.

My Lord, you are a just and giving God and I thank you for keeping me on this, your narrow path. Lord and I thank you for blessing me at each turn of my journey to health. As it comes you handle it.

Lord I trust in you, for I know, you have studied my needs and have seen fit to place me in the hands of my Oncologist Dr. John Link. Have your way Lord.

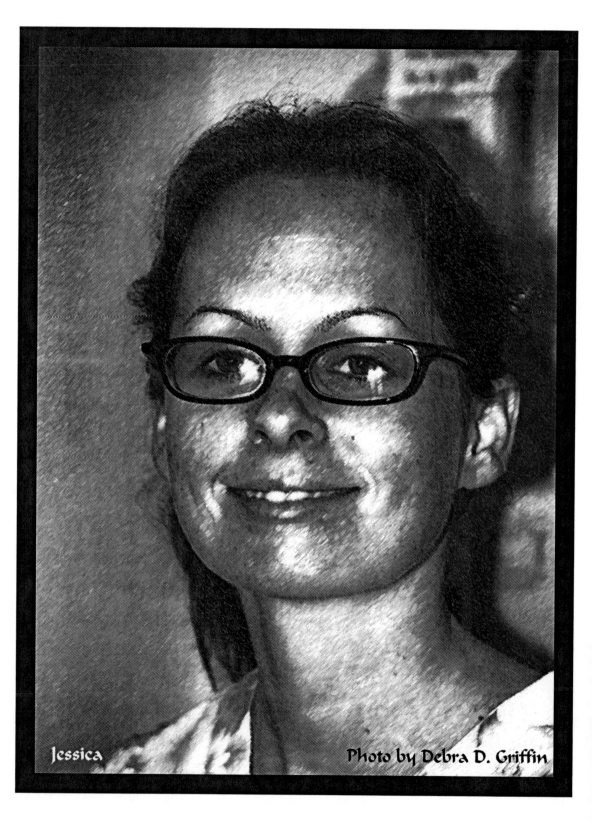

After I was examined by Dr. Link, Ree and I met with him in his office, where the three of us came up with a plan of action. The next 20 or so weeks would be be filled with lots of Chemo, scanning and more Chemo. Radiation would be looked at on a later date if Link felt it necessary. Dr. Link wanted to have my breast and underarm re-scanned. He also ordered full body and bone scans.

When our meeting with Link was over we were taken down the hall and introduced to Jessica who took my blood pressure, temperature, and weight.

Next I was taken to the Chemo room. There I met Lisa, the Registered Chemo Nurse. She made a genuine effort to comfort me as she explained the procedures.

A woman named Sandra drew my blood and they tested it right on the spot. After the results were in Lisa began administering the Chemo drugs.

I sat in a reclining chair and as the red drugs filled my veins, memories of Dorothy and her Chemotherapy brought a certain fear to me. It was then that I could almost hear her voice saying, "It's going to be alright." Ree held my hand.

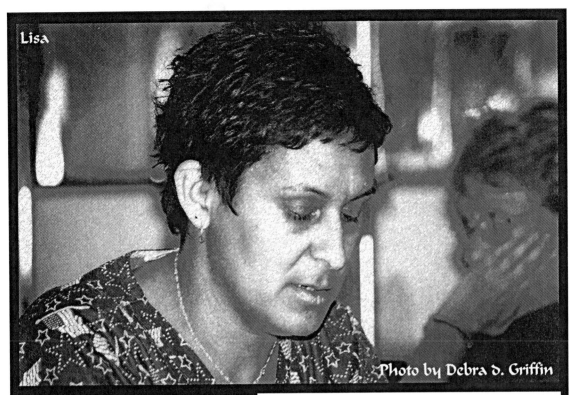

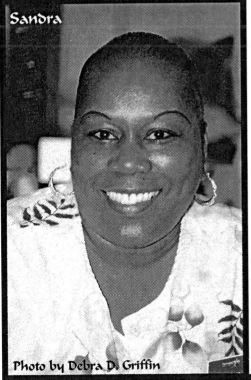

"Remember to drink lots of water. It will help keep your veins healthy," said Lisa.

"It will be easier on you and we will only have to stick you once."

"Yeah, but it won't keep me from coming back," I thought to myself.

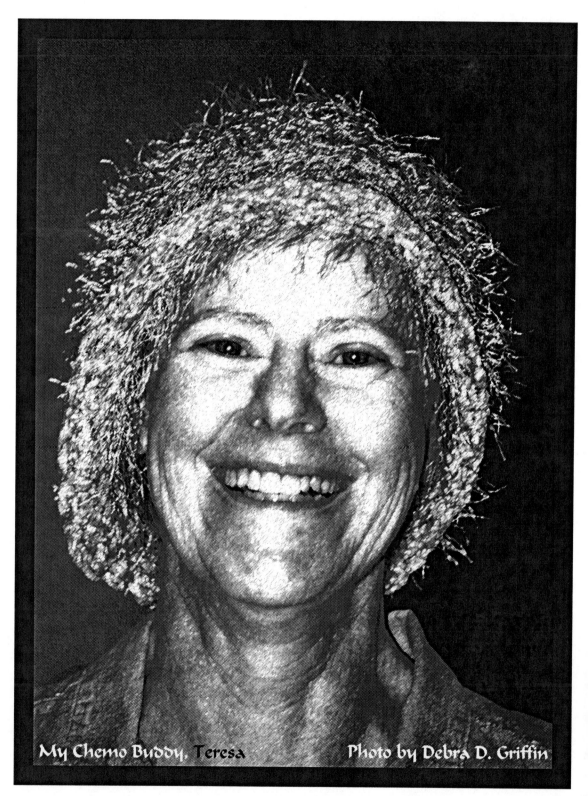

My Chemo Buddy, Teresa — Photo by Debra D. Griffin

The first re-scan of the breast and underarm showed that the cancer had metastasised to a lymph-node. The full body and bone scans showed cancer in the liver as well, there were two 2 cm tumors found.

Doctor Link assured me that at this point, wherever they found cancer, the Chemo would take care of it. "Don't worry, you have a good chance at beating this," are the words I let rock me to sleep at night.

These kind and gentle words also guided me into the Chemo room where I could always find hope waiting for me in the eyes of my Chemo buddies.

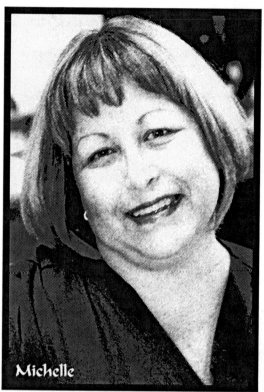
Michelle

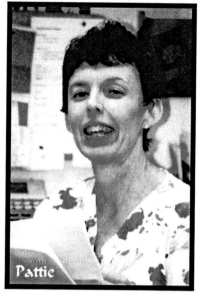
Pattie

Link's Girls

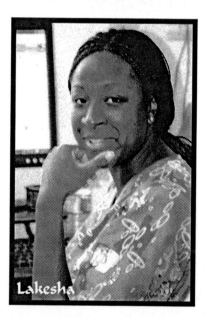
Lakesha

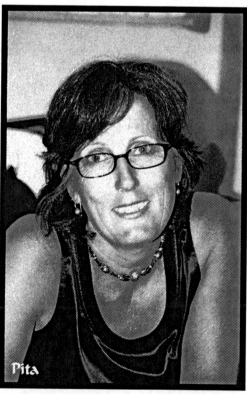
Pita

Photos by Debra D. Griffin

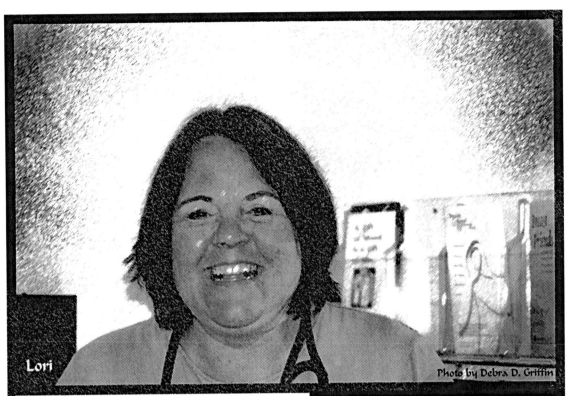

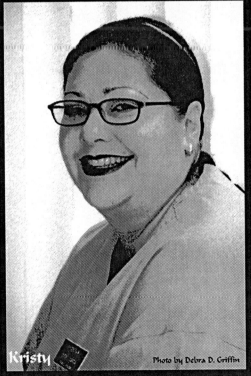

Where is my hope?
My hope is in your smiles.
Where does my strength come from?
Your smiles girls, your smiles.
And just why do you think I keep coming back?
Right, your smiles.
I am collecting smiles.

"my hair"

Debra D. Griffin

Photo by Marla D. Mitchell

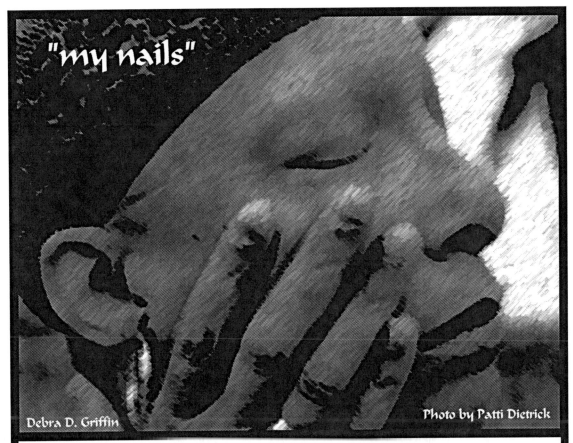

"my nails"

Debra D. Griffin — Photo by Patti Dietrick

Chemo, you are the thief that keeps on taking, you have taken my hair, my nails, and the strength from my bones.

Chemo, you are a travel agent, you have sent me pack'n with a one way ticket to menopause.

Lord, I need some clarification. I need the wisdom to understand. Lord tell me how is it that something that treats me so wrong can be so right for me.

...And Lord when do I get my hair back?

"I survived"

Debra D. Griffin

Photo by Patti Dietrick

I survived Chemo! Just when it started to feel that it held me down for the last count, the bell at the end of round two went off and I was standing on my feet. The Victor.

Fifteen years after the death of my sweet sister Dorothy, and to the date. I was given a reprieve. The Chains of cancer were no more and the sweet smell of victory was on my breath.

And yeah, I stood baldheaded, thin and weak, but I stood cancer free. You go God! You rock!

"Remission"

Debra D. Griffin

Photo by Patti Dietrick

With the fresh melodic sound of remission resounding through my being I found my self dancing the Jig. Theme music is what I needed. The absolute perfect pitch of peace-of-mind, Let me say it again. Remission.

Maybe once more as I have to ready myself for tomorrow. Remission.

Once more, for tomorrow always brings more decisions in this chorusline.
Remission, Remission Remission!

Well tomorrow did bring another decision. Reconstruction? To reconstruct or not to reconstruct was an awfully big question. When Dorothy had her mastectomy I never heard her talking about reconstruction. The idea of rebuilding a breast is a new phenomenon to me. So, I took this medicine real slow. Don't get me wrong, I liked the idea. But, for me it was deciding on how much of my decision would based on vanity or how much of this was totally necessary.

I had to take this one to the river of Jordan and pray.

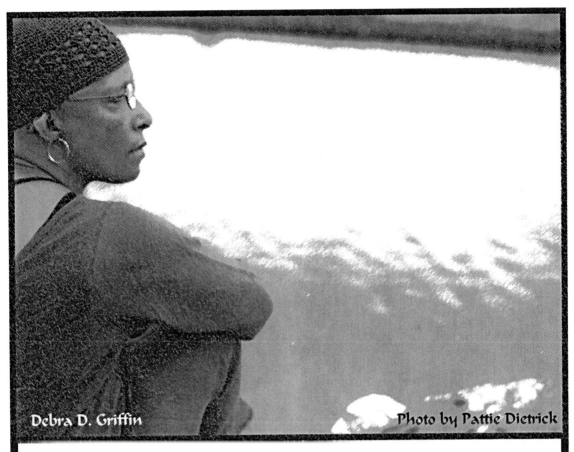
Debra D. Griffin
Photo by Pattie Dietrick

Here I am again Lord. Father I come to you today with a bowed head and a humble heart. God I am seeking wisdom. Help me Lord Jesus to make an intelligent decision concerning reconstruction. Lord I ask that you look beyond my faults and see my needs. Amen.

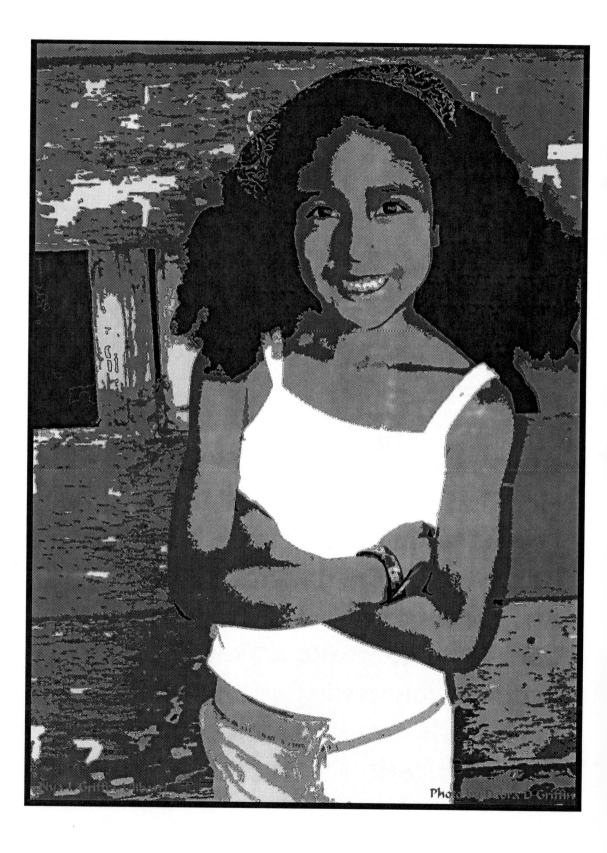

When people see me they comment on how strong they think I am, but at times I struggle in this thing. Most of the time I stumble on my answers. Like, which road will lead me to health with the least amount of resistance? Have I set realistic goals and will I be satisfied with the outcome? These are just a few of the questions I ask myself. Are they the right set of questions for sustaining life?

After surviving Chemo I'm scared to make the wrong decisions, decisions that may cause further damage or perhaps death.

And you, if asked to give up your breast, could you do it? Would you be swayed by one new opinion over another? Could you endure the physical pain? Will you live?

One morning I awoke with my answers. I took one look at Nya, my grand-daughter, and my answers I found in her smile.

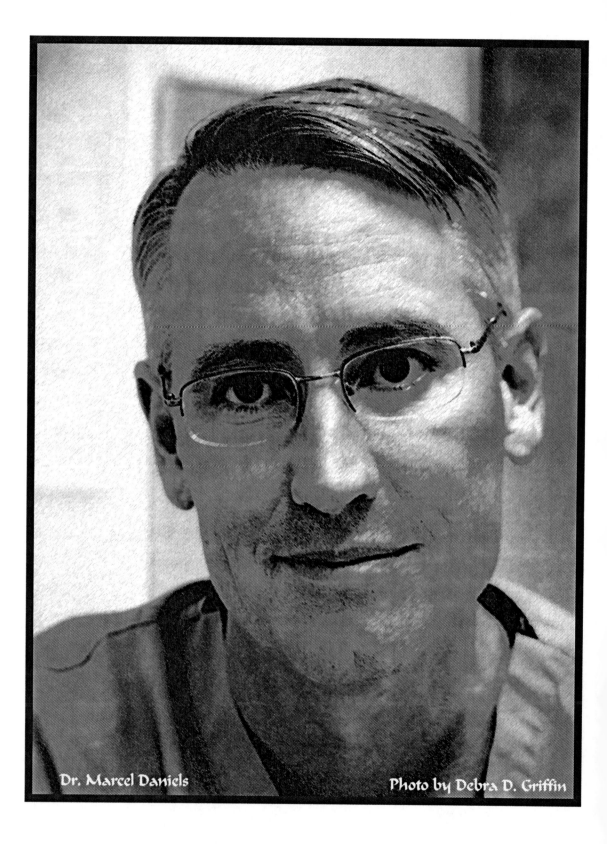

Dr. Marcel Daniels, a Plastic Surgeon, was recommended quite highly by Dr. Evans to perform my reconstruction surgery directly following the bi-lateral mastectomy. I was then forewarned about his sense of humor. If memory serves me, the phrase healthy dose was used to describe him. I thought to myself that a little levity would be a good thing. But what I found was a brilliant man overdosing on slapstick verity based antics. I liked him.

We spoke on several occasions leading up the point when we were ready to schedule the surgeries.

Time was getting short and as the first phase of my anticipated surgeries were being planned, Dr. Daniels began outlining the procedure. First the mastectomy and then reconstruction. My natural breasts would be removed and an expander would be put into place. The expander could then be filled with saline solution to create a mound, which would stretch the remaining skin allowing him to create the desired size. At that point implants could be emplaced. This would take several visits over many weeks.

But time did prevail and my surgery was scheduled.

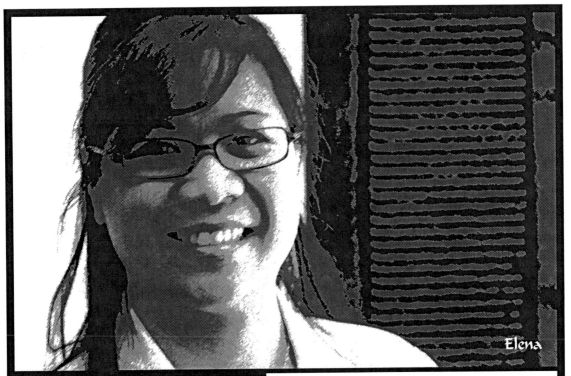

Elena

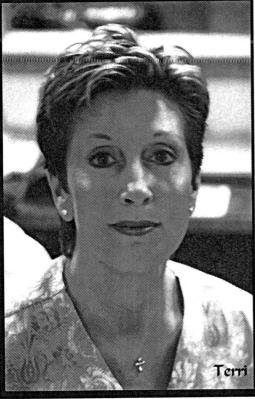

Terri

Thank-you, when ever I see chocolate Kisses or Hugs I will forever think of you. There is a little thing I like to say when bidding a fond farewell. "Be Sweet" and you have been just that. Sweet.

Photos by Debra D. Griffin

A Fact Untold

Rock

Photo by Debra D. Griffin

Rock, my sister's friend, brought this fact to my attention after reading my journal. I have not addressed a major issue in my writings. So, after giving it a lot of thought I am now ready to expose my dirty little secret. I am a smoker.

I have smoked since high school and regardless of whether I am currently physically puffing on a cigarette or not, I am a smoker. I am a time bomb waiting to happen and I am mentally smoking now as I type these words.

I use to think that if cancer were to happen to me I would be able to drop smoking like a bad habit. I think most smokers probably think the same or somewhere there a bouts. But nothing comes that easy in life, this applies to all bad vices.

Even though I wanted to quit and needed to quit, quitting just didn't happen for me with out a fight. My surgeons told me I could not have the surgeries until I was nicotine free. On again off again became my battle. I have, however, been able to quit and am now ready for the next phase. Surgery.

And although I am not currently smoking the effects of it on my body and my life will be affected for my forever. But, for now I just have to struggle and wait to see the payoffs.

Sisters

As you well know I did not choose you,
but if I did you would be exactly the same.

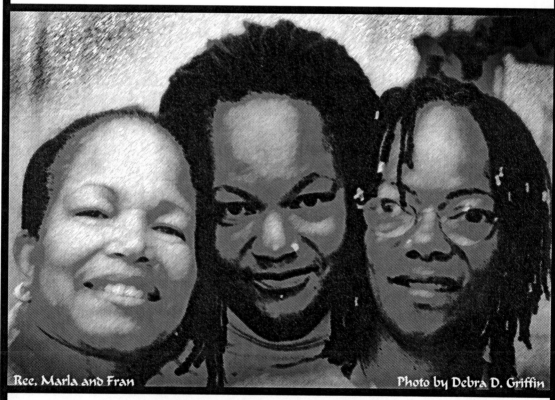

Ree, Marla and Fran

Photo by Debra D. Griffin

A part of my whole.

Well my day in surgery came soon enough. In fact maybe a little to soon as I hadn't worked through a major issue, fear. I was petrified. Panic completely took over and my ability to reason soundly collided with my need to express the terror.

That poor little nurse, all she was trying to do was get me to take off my jewelry...and I wasn't having it. You would have thought she was trying to take my first-born.
The thing that saved her was my sisters were able to calm me down. I wish I could bottle them up and sell them. Imagine you could whip out a can of SISTAH and your enemies, calm.

I don't remember anything else, not even drugs being administered. So I guess you could safely say that fear was my drug of choice that day.

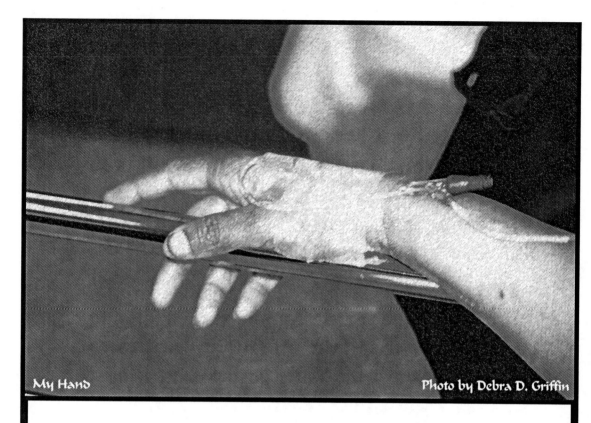

My Hand Photo by Debra D. Griffin

I feel another prayer come on my sistahs.

I feel the need to communicate with the Lord.

I feel the hunger for grace and salvation.

... And I feel it way down deep in my veins?

The pain following the surgery was off the Rictor Scale. Morphine, Vicodin and Darvocet became new additions to my vocabulary...and instant friends. I had no problems calling on them for relief.

Let me reiterate. I don't remember much about my surgery. However, I am able to recall my cousins' visits. I woke up from a fog and I saw Denise and Rhonda greeting my sisters. Jennifer came later. I wanted a prayer from her, but I can't seem to remember hearing her pray.

I was scheduled to be in the hospital for a couple of days but I got sick to my stomach and I was retained for two more days.

One or more of my sisters were constantly with me. Fran or Marla slept over each night. They slept on a rickety old cot in the corner next to my bed and both complained of back pain the next morning. I love them.

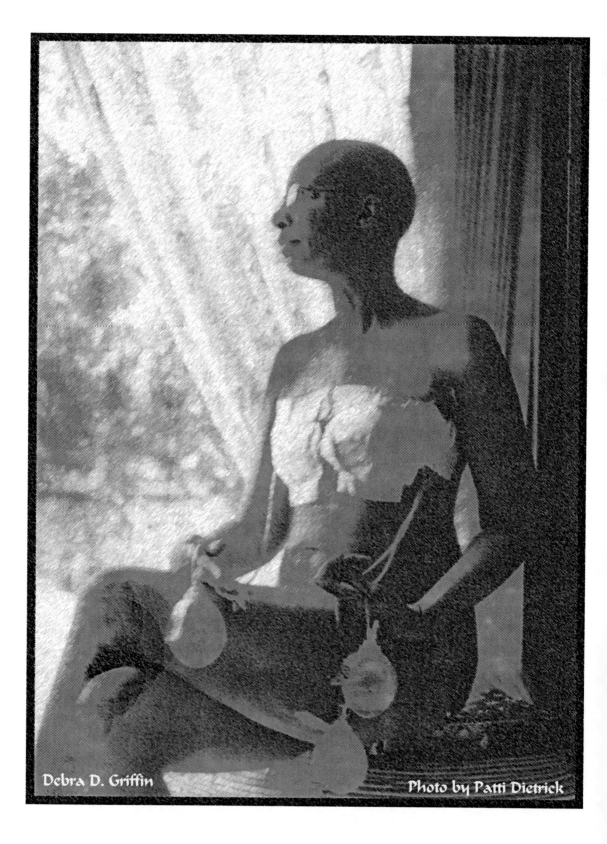

The morning I was released from Long Beach Memorial Hospital, Fran took me to visit with Dr. Daniels for my follow-up appointment. He said I was doing well (somebody had to tell me) and he gave some advise on aftercare and asked me to return the following week.

After the appointment Fran took me to Ree's house. It was there that I convalesced.

I learned a lot about my sisters during this time. I suppose you could say that the major thing I learned is they do not falter when they are called on for help.

While I lay convalescing a phrase that I heard years ago kept popping into mind. "If you want to know who your friends are just get in a situation where you can't take care of yourself and watch them run," So I took the time to really look at it as it pertained to my life's situation.

What I found absolutely astonished me! I am loved. I knew that, I just didn't have any idea to what degree. Oh, and I do have a host of family and friends that did run, they ran to me.

There were both friends and family running around taking care of my every need. They took me back and forth to my doctors appointments (which is a 70 mile trek), they fed me, they cleaned up after me and bathed me.

Yes, I did say bathed me.

Nya my 8 yr. old grand-daughter and her 10 yr. old best friend Jordan literally put me into a tub, lathered me up and bathed me. Never have I been witness to such a kindness. You should have been there to witness for yourself, such a gentle sweet kindness, as they dried, lotion and dressed this ailing old fart, me.

As the girls instructed me to raise my arms or reposition my feet, they spoke to me in a voice a mother uses when speaking to her infant. This touched my being all the way into the spirit, that place where only God goes. The Soul.

I must tell you that I was compliant. I know this because they gave me cookies and let me watch them play video games.

Oddly enough about this time my taste buds started to kick into gear. The first time I could really taste something was weeks ago when my cousin Denise cooked salmon for me. Now I was able to really enjoy food. My nails, blackened from the Chemo, were clearing up and there was hair on my head popping-up from the follicles.

I was healing quickly and was able to spend some time enjoying my good friends Liz, Shelly and Mac. Liz would come for me, and dinner and a movie seemed to be the thing I liked best. Shelly and I scrap booked and played dice games on her balcony for hours.

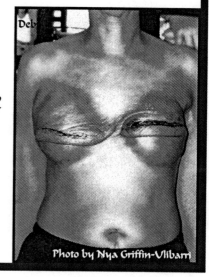

Photo by Nya Griffin-Ulibarri

Surprisingly the results of the surgery were remarkable and to my liking. I had seen many of this type of surgeries while I was doing my research on the web. Most, in my opinion, looked like hatchet jobs, giving the appearance that the set of breast couldn't possibly belong to anyone other than Frankenstein's Bride.

This was most important to me because, after all, I am an otherwise reasonably healthy young woman and single as well.

And dare I say, that I was eager to get the pumping started.

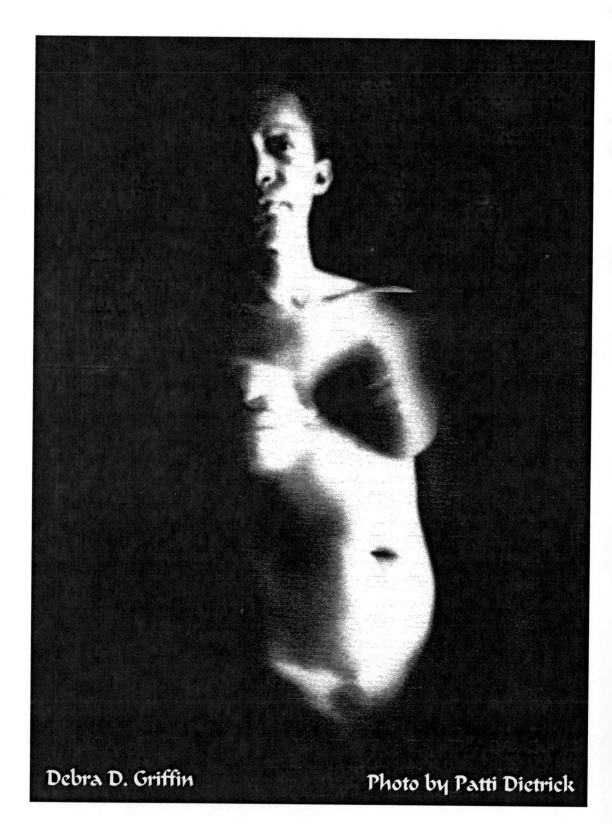

Piece of cake, let the pumping begin! Ha, so I thought. I soon learned that this wasn't to be the case.

The expander had some sort of magnetic device which had a portal, when found a needle could be inserted through my flesh and into it. Then a saline solution could be used to inflate it's bulb. I returned faithfully each week receiving approximately 80cc at each visit. It was on or about the sixth week I could not get out of my car and go into Dr. Daniels office. I sat for about thirty or so minutes just crying. I had endured enough. Dr. Daniels agreed and gave me a month off to prepare for phase two.

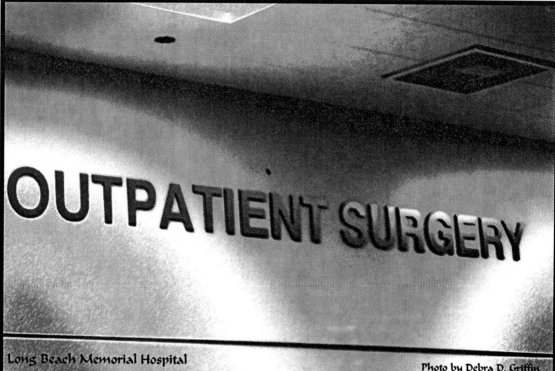

Long Beach Memorial Hospital — Photo by Debra D. Griffin

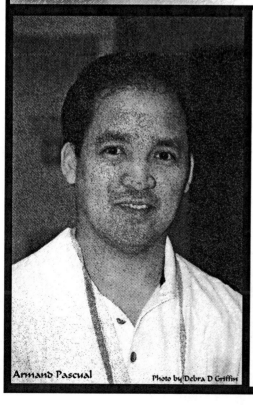

Armand Pascual — Photo by Debra D Griffin

Phase two of my breast reconstruction was done in Outpatient Surgery.

I couldn't believe I would be in good enough shape to be sent home in just a few hours.

This unsettled me and once again fear set in. The nursing staff did their best to soothe me.

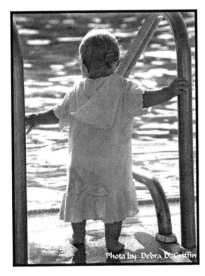

But fear will have you feeling like a baby too close to the water edge. It will totally immobilize you to the point where you can't move. I know I've talked about this before but this issue popped-up once again prior to my second surgery.

Dr. Daniels had to come out of the operating room just minutes before my surgery was to begin when he was informed about my behavior.

"Are you having surgery today," he asked. The way he delivered this question in that stone cold voice full of disapproval was enough for me to pull it together.

With the second surgery successfully behind me I lay half consciences and oblivious to the world. It took some time to recognize where I was and for that matter to figure out my sister's location. Wasn't it Ree who brought me here? I didn't ponder that long because Ree's face showed at the end of that thought like a period.

Ree gathered my things and helped me to dress. We were given the doctor's orders and the nurse wheeled me to the curb. Ree swung her car around to pick me up. The nurse helped me into the car and off we went. Destination Ree's.

At Ree's I slept for days. Exhausted.

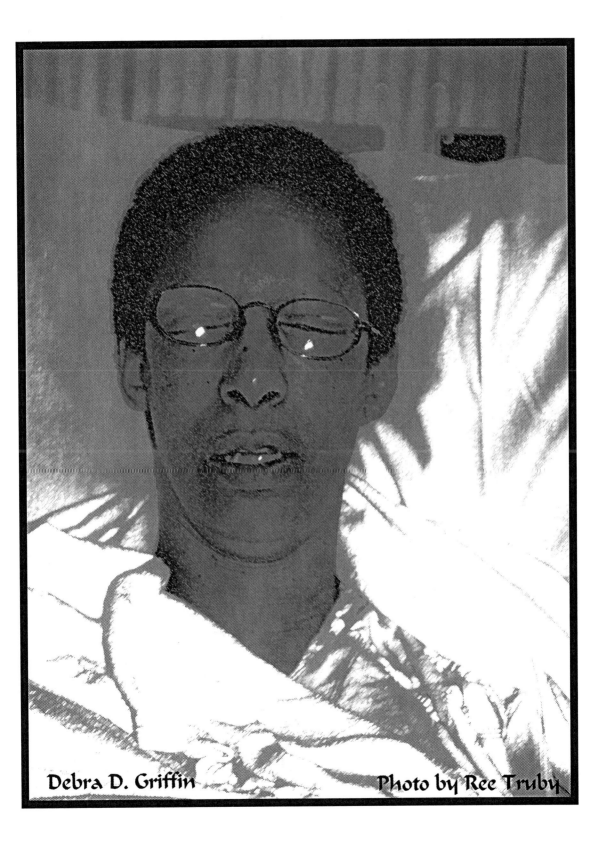

A Test of Strength

Debra D. Griffin

Tanya Griffin-Ulibarri

Things were going quite well for me. Sweet. I was making plans to attend my family reunion held this year in San Francisco, Ca. The hotel, air fares and reunion fees all paid. All I was waiting on was my departure date to arrive.

But two weeks before the time I was scheduled to leave I noticed a scab growing the left breast. When the scab fell there was a small hole exposing the implant. I called Dr. Daniel and he ordered an emergency surgery to remove the implant and repair the skin.

A set back, just a test of strength.

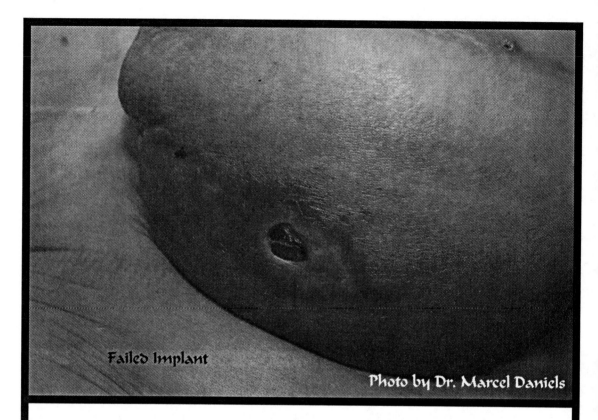

Failed Implant

Photo by Dr. Marcel Daniels

I am a very optimistic person, hope driven. it is just my nature. So forgive me if I seem have a tendency to minimize the pain in all this. It just wasn't until my left implant failed that my world came crushing down in on me. Boom!

But Once the gates were opened I began to focus on all my feelings. Then could I see the many disappointing issues surrounding my disease, recovery and my financial status. Believe me it was a very saddening and sobering time.

As I became more concerned about the effects of the disease, rather than the disease itself, a feeling of helplessness overtook me and I became an emotional wreck. My doctor promised I could go if things got better, and as God would have it.

I was on that plane with my family and healed enough to attend and enjoy the reunion. There, I took this picture off my great-nephew Garrett and my grand-baby Nya. Garrett is her most favorite cousin in the whole wide world.

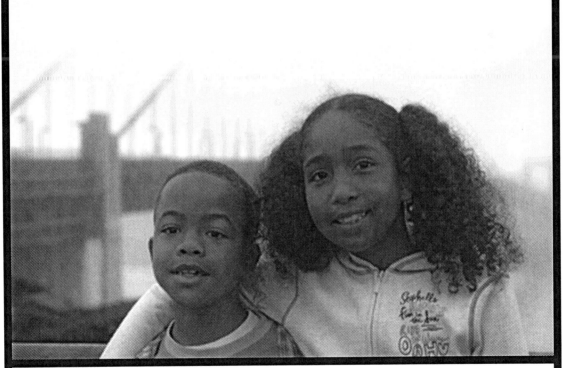

Garrett and Nya In of front the Goldengate Bridge

Love, Music, and the Angels Who Watch Over Me

Love

For centuries (or more simply put, since the beginning of time) masters, philosophers, scientists and/or just great thinkers have tried to pinpoint the meaning of love. The question thus far and remains, "What is it?"

Well, I won't bother to liken myself to the for-mention master minds, but I do want to show you what it means to me.

Several months ago I was standing in line in Ralph's Market...tired, bald and scalp gleaming like a beacon. Behind me stood a strawberry blond boy. He was just more than a toddler. He was sandwiched between me and his mother's cart. All of a sudden I felt two little arms embrace my legs. I looked down into the face of this smiling angel. At first I thought maybe he had gotten confused and wasn't paying attention, perhaps he thought I was his mom for a split second. Then, a moment later I heard his mother ask him, "Why did you hug that lady?" He answered only to say, "Just because, because I love her". This is what love means to me and how I want to love. "JUST BECAUSE"

Music

Today I am reminded of a song entitled, "Music Saved My Life," by Christina Gaudet. It is off her DANCE IN THE WIND album. It makes me wonder how anyone can get along without music. For me, music is in the air and should be taken in with each breath.

I was just recently asked how I made it through chemotherapy as though it was some God awful tragedy. My answer was simply this: "I don't remember much about the chemo, what I do remember is the MUSIC." You see my daughter Tammera and Dr. L.R. Strom, (our family friend) bought me an iPod for my birthday. I began to take it everywhere with me. I was plugged into it constantly, and it soon became my saving grace. Especially with each blood test and the wait for the results...most definitively soon as I knew I would be given chemo the headphones went on and the music, it filled my soul.

As luck would have it, even now I don't remember many things about the chemo, but I do remember the beautiful music for it truly saved my life.

The Angels Who Watch Over Me

"I believe with everything I am that there are angels living amongst us, right here on earth...sent to comfort, to aide, to teach and to protect."

I also believe that during my battle with cancer God sent me such angels to guide and watch over me and I will forever be filled to the brim with gratitude. Surely given the way I feel about this subject I would totally be remised if I didn't take the time to pay homage to my angels at this time.

The first angel came to me by surprise as he is a musician I have admired for many years. I truly am in awe of his showmanship and his mastery of his craft. I was sitting at a table minding my own business during a Newport Jazz Party event. Engaged in a conversation with my sister Ree and a few of our friends. We were speaking on the topic of love. I had just reminded my sister of the quote our father often used. "Never let the sun go down on someone you love." I believe and took this to mean that one must never neglect to let a person know they are loved. In passing I also mentioned after noticing that Mr. Lewis Nash, a masterful drummer had taken the stage...how much I did revere him. Well, today Lewis is my brother and one of my life's greatest treasures. God!

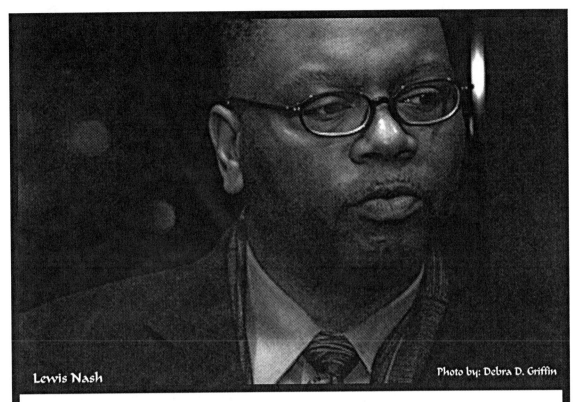

Lewis Nash Photo by: Debra D. Griffin

Debra - Thought you might like this....

Saturday, February 17, 2007 – Service
"Life's most persistent and urgent question is, 'What are you doing for others?'"
~Martin Luther King, Jr.~

Today's Affirmation
I am open to new ways of serving others.

Today's Meditation
Dear God,
Thank You for opening my eyes to unseen opportunities to serve those souls around me.
You have placed me in a world where I am in frequent contact with my brothers and sisters.
We are here to love one another.
We are here to serve one another.
Let my life exemplify that love and service toward others.
Thank You, God.
Amen

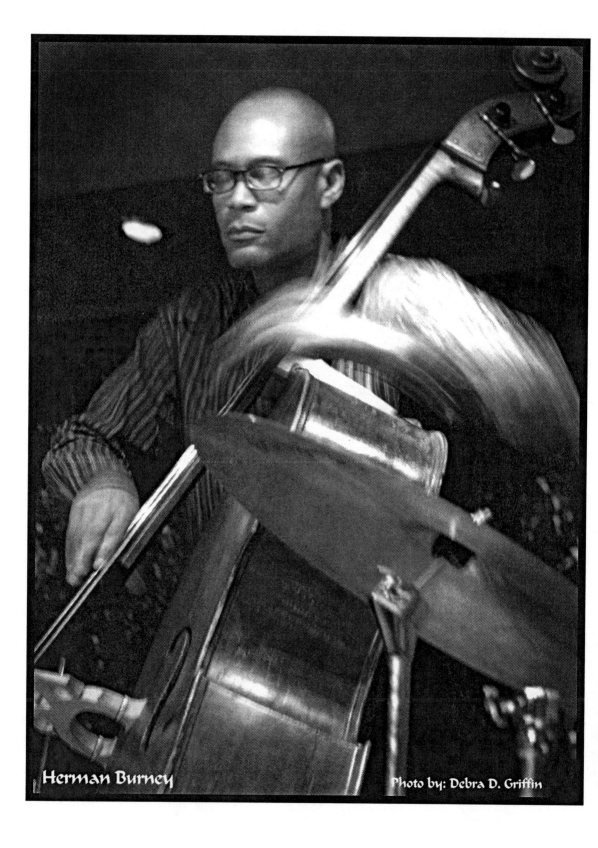

I was a bit more prepared for this next angel who entered my life. Although I had never set eyes on this gentleman before I heard him play during a cruise aboard the Oosterdam I knew he was mine. I did recognize the halo and I was mesmerized both by his divine light and the upright bass he was making love to.

The Lord did say to make a joyful noise and this young man's music did feed my hunger like food for the soul. Oh what joyous melodies did nourish my heart and I could hardly wait to tell him so. After the show had ended I marched up to the stage with my sister Ree in tow and unloaded my hearts contents. Herman Burney, my "babe brotha" was born to me that evening and I will indeed cherish this gift that the Lord has given me.

God is so good to me! Seems as though wherever I turned there was love waiting on me. Even when I look back on those times when my health was at its weakest stages the picture I see is a very hopeful and loving one. Full of many surprises!

And so this next angel as she was not a surprise to me the reason she was sent absolutely blew me away! Ms. Holly Hofmann, the finest flautist the world will ever know, is my sister survivor. I wrote Holly a brief note after attending one of her performances, because I was touched in a way that I had never been touched. I literally felt the healing properties in her music. I tell you, music saved me.

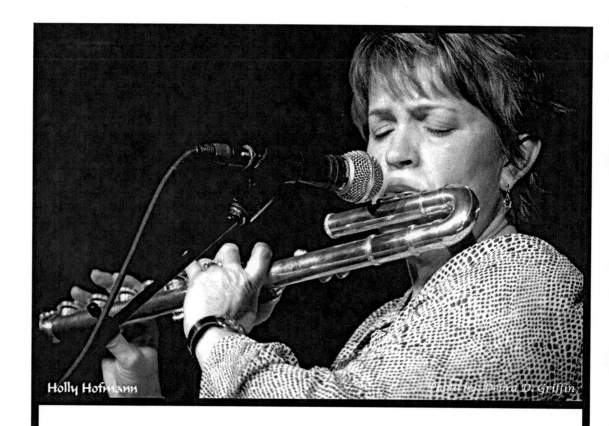

Holly Hofmann

Heal me

Touch me with your music,
heal me with thine song.
Let your heart's contents
flow through me,
'til the Lord's work is done.

There were many other angels to follow and I found them in the most unbelievable places. Like, MySpace. That's right, I am on MySpace...hit me up. I am at: MySpace.com/serious1cancer.

One day when I was fighting a bad case of cabin fever and while surfing the net I blue crushed right into this beautiful cyber world. Once there I found many wonderful friends, survivor sisters, organizations for breast cancer survivors, Christians warriors and, to my surprise, family.

I mean, sisters, daughters, sons, nieces, nephews...I found them ALL and not a one of them had ever mentioned that they had spots on the space. The feeling of being sick and shut in has never been further from me and loneliness has never darkened my door again. I can always find someone to talk to, pray or laugh and cry with. Life is good and I am holding on to it!!!

Metastatic Disease

I learned a new medical term today, "Metastatic Disease." I was sitting at my desk minding my own business...nothing new as this is an everyday occurrence, and where I find solace. I was working on having a new web site built by my friend from D.C. Mr. Joe Perry

However, on this day I found myself struggling to do the simple tasks I usually do blind folded. This day, I found myself repeating the same mistakes over and over. I could not remember what I had just done from this moment to the next. A sense of frustration like no other overtook me and anxiety roared through me only to add to the confusion that was mounting. Fear sent me roaming the house dazed in search of help.

In the living room I found my daughter Tammera, cousin Sukari, Suki (as I fondly call her) was braiding Tammera's hair. I desperately tried to convey to Tammera what was going on as she looked on in horror. "Mom are you kidding me?" she asked. Which enraged me as I am the mother and she the child and no matter how grown she thought she was....blah, blah.

In the emergency room, (I was taken there because they thought I was having a stroke) when I became coherent...I over heard the doctor talking to my family about brain metastasis. He said it was common with metastatic disease. Oh my, it's back!

The next few days were filled with doctors, testing, and the suggestion of gamma rays. They call it Gamma Knife Surgery. I was referred to Dr. Duma, who, I was told was the leading doctor in this field. I was also told I was a good candidate for this procedure.

Once home I put a call in for a prayer vigil to have my angels on MySpace to pray for me. The prayers came to me in a steady flow. I was able to make my decision to have the procedure done after talking to my daughters, sisters and my online angel "Kim is beating stage 4 breast cancer for 2 years."

After the Gamma Knife surgery I was again seen by Dr. Duma. His good news soothed my ailing heart as his findings put me back into remission. Thank you Lord, thank you!!!

Later in the week I Spoke to Herman Burney and was I able to express my feelings on gratitude so feverishly that it inspired an original composition, a song in ode to me. It is entitled "Grounded in Gratitude." I like that!!!

I also decided to continue on with reconstruction. As the implant needed to be replaced after its failure just months ago. Yes, this meant a dorsal flap, another expander and implant replacement.

Bring it on! I'm holding on to the words, clean scan!!!

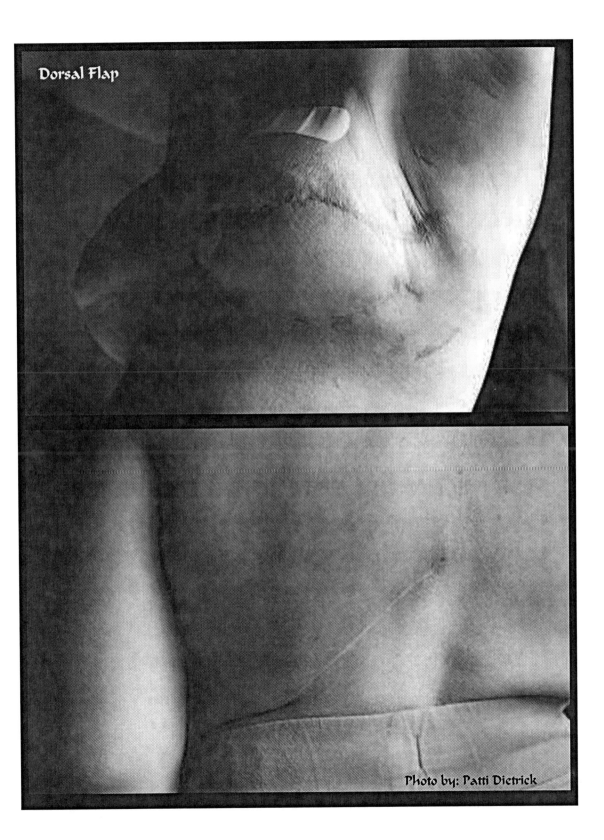

"At some point in life we all will encounter a time when we must stop and take stock in our inventories. Now for some I am sure this will mean the tangible possessions, which were acquired through monetary riches. However, for others like myself, this will mean the emotional treasures that love, respect, integrity and honor have made priceless."

Debra D. Griffin

Now with all that said and out of the way, let me take stock of my inventories. The most important thing is that I have taken two more PET/CT scans since last mentioned, and both show no evidence of the disease. Hallelujah! Go ahead and give God his props. Next, and although the failed implant was a set back it was not life threatening and will heal in time.

As I am sure you can imagine cancer is a very expensive disease to fight, but as long as there is breath in this body I can work. With work there is possibility for prosperity and I plan to be going back and rejoining my old crew as soon as I am able. Soon.

Last, but not least, my girls are doing quite well. Jessica is working everyday in Arizona. Tammera runs her own company, Tye is on the mend and my Sisters still love me.

Oh yeah, Liz has a new grand-baby, a girl. Welcome to life Zakiah Michatu Sesay.

The Passionist Community

650 Sheppard Avenue East, Toronto, Ontario

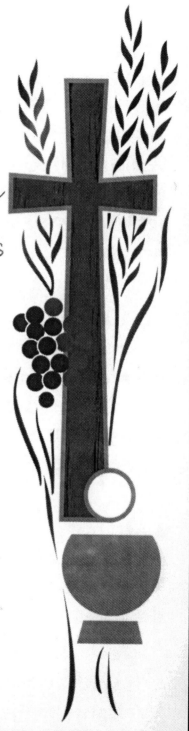

<u>Deborah Griffen's Special Intentions</u> will share perpetually in the benefit of daily Mass, of other Masses and prayers offered in every Passionist Monastery, and in the apostolic works of the Passionist Missionaries.

Father Rector, C.P.

Requested by

<u>Bill & Naomi Stephens</u>
<u>with love and prayers</u>

Date: <u>March 15, 2006</u>

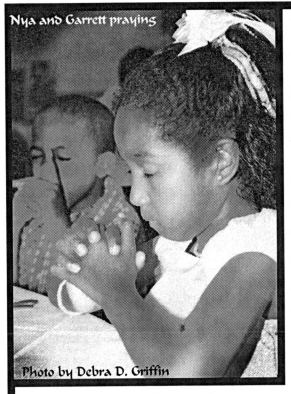

Nya and Garrett praying

Photo by Debra D. Griffin

I never asked why me, I rather ask, why not me? This disease took the life of my sister Dorothy and I am not any better than she. Cousin Van says that God isn't finished with me yet. I believe it was the prayers of the many believers that saved me. From the first day I was diagnosed there were prayers. In fact, that evening my younger cousin Jennifer Arthur prayed for me over the phone. Kristen Truby, my niece, prayed and continues to keep me in the light of prayer. My grand-baby prayed. A church in Canada sent me a Declaration of Prayer. It wasn't until days later that I realized who I knew in Canada. Bill & Naomi Stephens, my friend Shannon's parents, I met them briefly when I photographed their family's visit to the O.C. Aunt Carolyn's Church kept me on their prayer list until I went into remission, then they put me on their praise list.

As the hours approach, the third and final surgery...it became time to reflect on all my issues concerning the past events. Carefully perusing all matters, I first discovered I have not yet lay claim or ownership to the mounds that I will in the near future refer to as my breasts. Will a nipple make the difference?

Secondly, damages caused by the surgeries and Chemotherapy, can they be corrected or will I just adapt? Will I forever have these scanty tresses or will my hair be thick enough to cover my big head? Those who know me, know I need a healthy set of bangs to hide my mighty forehead. Will my brainpower be restored? Will I ever verbally be able put two sentences together without struggling for the correct words? Chemo does kill off brain cells.

Oh and finally, how will I fit back into my old life? Although I am the same person my abilities have changed. My general outlook on life has changed. Hopefully for the better.

At this point, I must say good-bye to you and bid you a fond farewell. For I can not take you with me on the next phase of my journey. You see, I strongly believe that this next surgery will make me whole and as a woman I will need some privacy.

But I do have a few more thoughts to share with you:

Hold yourself.
Be your own advocate.
Walk in the light of prayer.
Seek knowledge and make your decisions wisely.
Smile and keep a lot of smiling faces around you.

Remember that God has a plan for you and when ever you take one step he will take two. Be Sweet!

Glossary

Glossary

Arteriosclerosis - a group of diseases characterized the thickening and loss of elasticity of the arterial walls occurring in three forms, atherosclerosis, Monckberg's arteriosclerosis, and arteriolosclerosis.

Breast Friends - a peer support and mentoring program for newly diagnosed breast cancer patients, sponsored by Memorial Care Breast Center at Long Beach.

Breast Reconstruction - is a surgical procedure to recreate the contour of the breast, using either prosthesis or your own tissues.

Chemotherapy - treatment of disease by chemical agents.

Core Biopsy - or core needle biopsy, is a percutaneous procedure that involves removing small samples of breast tissue using a hollow "core" needle.

Cyst Aspiration - or aspiration biopsy uses a needle to draw cells or fluid from the cyst.

EECP Therapy - (Enhanced External Counterpulsation Therapy) is a treatment that enhances the circulation to all organs of the body. It does this by squeezing the blood from the peripheral lower extremities back to the heart. Then the heart can send oxygen to the lungs to feed the body.

Expander - is an empty implant shell that inflates as fluid is injected into a port under the skin.

Invasive Ductal Carcinoma - a neoplasm arising from the duct epithelium of the breast that does not show preponderance of other histological features. This is the most common type of invasive breast cancer and accounts for approximately 70% of breast cancers.

Glossary (continued)

Mastectomy - excision of the breast. The two most commonly used types of mastectomy are called simple and modified radical. In both of these procedures; the chest muscle is not removed. As a result, the arm strength remains making it easier for reconstruction.

Metastasis - the transfer of disease from on organ or part of the body to another not directly connected with it, due either to transfer of pathogenic microorganisms or transfer of cells; all malignant tumors are capable of metastasizing.

PET/CT Scan - (Positron Emission Tomography/Computed Tomography) a PET scan can detect abnormalities in cellular activity generally before there is any anatomical change found with ultrasound, X-rays, CT or MRI. It can also distinguish between benign and malignant masses, where the above modalities can only confirm there is a mass.

Remission - diminution or abatement of the symptoms of a disease; the period where such diminution occurs.

Acknowledgments

Thank you

When I was in need,
you came for me.
You held my hand,
and you gave the thing
I needed the most.
A FRIEND!

Tammera J. Griffin & Antonio A. Ulibarri
Tynisha R. Griffin - Jessica R. Griffin
Revonia J. Truby and Family - Frances J. Hoxie and Family
Marla Denise Mitchell - Dorothy's Children and Grandchildren
David P. & Deborah L. Mitchell and Family
Tommie R. & Pong Yo Mitchell and Family
Roslind Bell and Family - Van L. & Merdice Coleman and Family
Mickael J. Coleman and Family - Aunt Carolyn and the Truby Clan
Thelma Mettoy - Eloisa Ridgely and Family - Patti Dietrick - Neil France
Kristin A. N. Truby - Herlinda R. Mitchell and Family - Jennifer Arthur
Denise Barnes - Rhonda Arthur - Marva Mitchell - Khafid A. Ibrahim
Azziza B. Ibrahim - Zainab B. Ibrahim - Marilyn Hughes - Florida Arthur
The California Mitchells - The Chicago Mitchells - The Howards
The Detroit Mitchells - Lawrence R. Strom - Gloria Ginyard
Roy Gilliam - Jessie Finley - Sukari and The Finley Clan - Denise Cooper
Altheal & Anthony Randolph - Craig & Shelly McDonald and Family
The Staff and friends at Ritz Camera Centers
Liz Valenzuela - Nicolas Koury - Alex - Cheryl - Michelle
Claire - Destiny - Robert - Rosie - Alexi - Marlene - Teresa
The Staff at Global Cardio Care - Dr. R. Weaver
Sara - Dean - Julie - Glinda - LaMar - Ben - Eric - Joey
Adrian - Louis - Josh
The Staff at GalaCare Medical Clinic - Dr. Fred Kyazze
Ree - Arcille - Veronica
The Staff at Breastlink - Dr. John Link
Jessica - Lisa - Sandra - Lori - Michelle - Pattie - Pita - Lakesha - Kristy
Long Beach Memorial Breast Center - Dr. Gretchen M. Stipec
LaJetta
Dr. Tomi Evans - Donna
Dr. Marcel Daniels - Elena - Terri
and a special thanks to: Long Beach City College - Dr. Pauline Merry
Nya I. Griffin-Ulibarri - Jordan Rozenek and Steven A. Wright

I acknowledge you and raise you up. For I know
it was your prayers and efforts that saved me.
Because, you bowed your heads and lifted me
into the light of prayer. I can utter these words:
By his stripes I am healed.

Resources

Resources

American Cancer Society
800-227-2345
www.cancer.org

American Society of Plastic Surgeons
800-635-0635
www.plasticsurgery.org

National Cancer Institute
Cancer Information Service
800-422-6237
www.nci.nih.gov

Y-ME National Organization
for Breast Cancer
800-221-2141
www.y-me.org

Breast Friends
MemorialCare Breast Center
Todd Cancer Institute
562-933-7815

Imani's
Breast Care
510-465-7333

Good Reading

NO LESS A WOMAN: Ten Women Shatter the Myths about
   Breast Cancer
      By: Deborah H. Kahane, M.S.W.

THE BREAST CANCER SURVIVAL MANUAL: A Step-by-Step Guide for
   the Woman with Newly Diagnosed Breast Cancer
      By: John Link, M.D.

THE RACE IS RUN ONE STEP AT A TIME
      By: Nancy Brinker

INVISIBLE SCARS: A Guide to Coping with the Emotional Impact of
   Breast Cancer
      By: Mimi Greenberg, Ph.D.

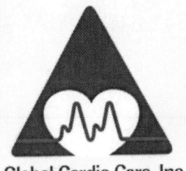

Sara Soulati
Founder & President

sara@globalcardiocareinc.com
mobile 949.697.5500

Global Cardio Care, Inc.

633 Aerick St. ♥ Inglewood, CA 90301 ♥ 310.412.8181
fax 310.412.9221 ♥ www.globalcardiocareinc.com

DATE OF SERVICE: 04/14/2004

CLINICAL INDICATION: Debra D. Griffin presented with Peripheral vascular disease.

PROCEDURE: EECP Treatment program consisting of 35 hours of therapy.

FINDINGS: Her peripheral augmentation of blood flow to her heart was approx. 15 percent. Throughout the course of her treatment she was able to increase that percentage to 60%, thus greatly affecting her circulation. In the process Ms. Griffin has lost a total of 72 lbs. and was able to quit smoking. To date she maintains healthy blood pressure and cholesterol levels.

Phone: (323) 566-6911
Fax (323) 566-6896

REVONIA TRUBY, RNP, MSN, PHN
OBGyn, Women's Health & Adolescent Medicine
Gala Care Medical Clinic

Suite 201
11905 So. Central Avenue
Los Angeles, CA. 90059

Date of Exam 4/19/2005

Diagnosis: Fibrocystic Breast disease:

1. Large asymmetric breast with multiple large cysts both breast. Left breast @ 4 o'clock hard fixed mass.

Plan:

1. Referral to Long Beach memorial Breast Center for diagnostic mammogram.
2. Referral to Dr. Tomi Evans, General Surgeon.
3. Referral to Dr. John Link, Oncologist.
4. Consider plastic surgeon.
5. Consider support systems.

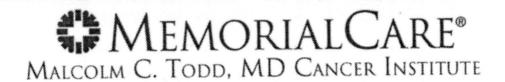

Gretchen M. Stipec, M.D.
Mammography, Breast Ultrasound
Intervention Procedures

Long Beach Memorial Breast Center
701 E. 28th Street, Suite 200
Long Beach, CA 90806
Phone: 562-933-7880
Fax: 562-933-7810

THE STANDARD OF EXCELLENCE IN HEALTH CARE

DATE OF REPORT: 04/29/2005

PREOPERATIVE DIAGNOSIS: Status post biopsy left lower outer quadrant approximately 4 cm mass, palpable.

SPECIMEN (S) Left breast lower outer quadrant, core biopsies.

MICROSCOPIC DESCRIPTION: The cores show replacement by infiltrating ductal carcinoma. There are large areas of central sclerosis. The tumor shows less than 10% open tubule formation and principally infiltrates as cords of highly malignant appearing cells. Mitotic activity is brisk and counted at 12 mitoses in 10 high power fields.

FINAL DIAGNOSIS: Invasive ductal carcinoma.
High grade, 8/9 (MBR score 3-9/9)

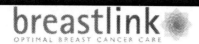

Dr John S. Link MD
President and Medical Director
Breast Medical Oncologist

Email link@breastlink.com, www.breastlink.com

Long Beach
701 E. 28th Street Suite 201
Long Beach, CA. 90806
562-933-7820 Fax 562-933-7819

Pacific Coast
3445 Pacific Coast Hwy Suite 220
Torrance, CA. 90505
310-539-2300 Fax 310-539-9185

Orange Coast
9900 Talbert Ave Suite 103
Fountain Valley, CA. 92708
714-378-5011 Fax 714-378-5051

Administration
23430 Hawthorne Blvd Suite 340
Torrance, CA. 90505
310-791-6610 Fax 310-791-6630

Breastlink Medical Group Inc.

DATE OF SERVICE: 05/19/2005

CLINICAL INDICATION: Newly diagnosed high nuclear grade invasive ductal carcinoma in the left breast with apparent axillary and liver metastases.

TREATMENT: Chemotherapy from May through October of 2005. Adriamycin/Cyclophosphamide, four cycles and Taxotere chemotherapy, twelve cycles.

FINDINGS: Complete disappearance of all cancer including liver metastases.

Fantastic attitude, pt continues to be disease free.

TELEPHONE
(562) 426-0338

FACSIMILE
(562) 427-4282

Women's Surgical Associates
Breast Specialists Medical Group, Inc.
Tomi Evans, M.D.
DIPLOMATE, AMERICAN BOARD OF SURGERY

DISORDERS OF THE BREAST
GENERAL AND LAPAROSCOPIC SURGERY

701 E. 28TH STREET, #411
LONG BEACH, CA 90806

DATE OF SURGERY: 12/08/2005

PREOPERATIVE DIAGNOSIS (ES): History of T3 N1 breast cancer with known liver metastasis. i.e. T4. Status post chemotherapy with a PET/CT scan showing complete resolution of all disease in all areas.

PROCEDURE (S):

1. Left modified radical mastectomy.
2. Right simple mastectomy.
3. Bilateral reconstruction with tissue expansion.

INDICATION (S): Ms. Griffin-Ibrahim is a 51 year-old African-American who presented with a large left breast mass laterally. Workup was consistent with a T3 N1 invasive ductal carcinoma. Unfortunately her PET/CT scan did show evidence of liver metastasis. She completed her extensive Adriamycin, Cytoxan, Taxotere chemotherapy. Her follow-up PET/CT has shown resolution of the disease in all areas; her breast, axilla and liver no longer show evidence of disease. Clinically she has very difficult breast exams with a lot of cystic change. The obvious firm mass found in the lower outer left breast has resolved. There is no longer palpable adenopathy. She has opted, knowing that she has had metastatic liver involvement to still go forward with bilateral mastectomies and tissue expansion reconstruction. She understands that there will be a discussion regarding the left breast for possible radiation therapy pending the outcome of today's pathology results.

I M A G E
Aesthetic & Reconstructive Surgery

562.597-4575
www.imagemd.com

Marcel F. Daniels, M.D., F.A.C.S., F.I.C.S.

DATE OF SURGERIES: 12/08/2005 (1st STAGE)
05/02/2006 (2nd STAGE)

PROCEDURES:

BILATERAL BREAST RECONSTRUCTION WITH EXPANDER (1st STAGE)
Reconstruction of both breasts with insertion of expanders under the chest wall skin and muscles.

BILATERAL BREAST RECONSTRUCTION WITH EXPANDER (2nd STAGE)
Removal of the breast expanders, create bilateral breast pockets and place permanent reconstructive breast implants.

BILATERAL CAPSULECTOMY (SUBPECTORAL REAUGMENTATION)
Removal of fibrous capsules surrounding the tissue expanders and replacement of implants in the subpectoral position.

Kenneth M. Tokita, M.D.
Radiation Oncologist
Medical Director
(949) 417-1100 / fax (949) 417-1165
Email: ktokita@ccoi.org

Cancer Center of Irvine

16100 Sand Canyon Avenue, Suite 130
Irvine, CA 92618
www.ccoi.org

DATE OF SERVICE: 4/21/2006

REFERRING PHYSICIAN: John Link, MD

CLINICAL INDICATION: Breast carcinoma/liver metastasis

COMPARISON: Prior PET Scan report dated 8/26/2005

PROCEDURE: Radiopharmaceutical: F-18 Deoxyglucose, 15 millicuries injected intravenously into the left antecubital fossa.

After the intravenous administration of F-18 Deoxyglucose, the patient underwent a standard 45-minute uptake phase. Subsequently, the patient was placed on a General Electric DST 16 slice PET CT scanner, and images were obtained from the vertex to the proximal thighs.

FINDINGS:

BRAIN: A dedicated brain study was not performed, but extracted images do not demonstrate asymmetries that would suggest neoplasm.

NECK AND CHEST: There are no hypermetabolic asymmetries within the lymph nodes of the neck or chest to suggest neoplasm. There are no FDG abnormalities in the lung parenchyma to suggest visceral disease.

ABDOMEN AND PELVIS: There is physiologic activity in the kidneys, ureters, bladder and gut. There is no evidence of neoplasm.

SKELETON: There are no focal abnormalities to suggest neoplasm.

IMPRESSION:

1. The scan findings do not suggest neoplasm.
2. No interval Change since the prior study dated 8/26/2005.

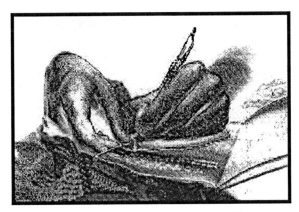

Illustration by Donna Osborn Clark

At the Author's request, 5% of each sale from
A Journey to Wellness: A Series of Collective Thoughts
will be grateful donated to:

Breast
Cancer
Care & Research
Fund

Printed in the United States
96458LV00002B/317-396/A